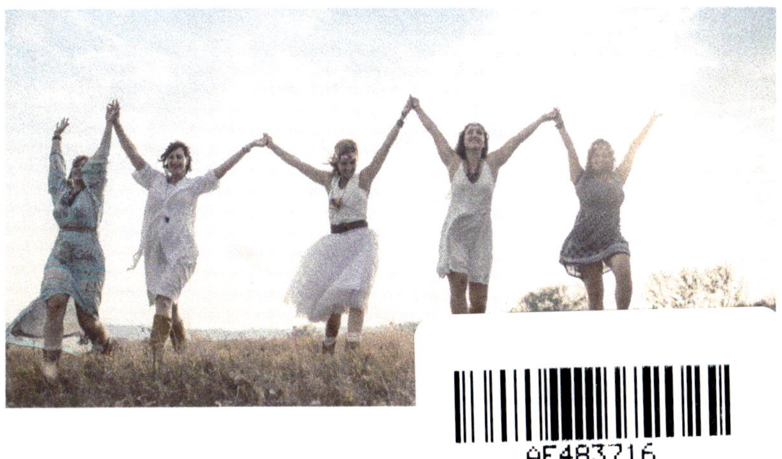

Introduction

I am so glad you're here.

If you are reading this, chances are you've started (or are considering starting) a GLP-1 medication and are ready for real, lasting change. First, I want you to know this: choosing to care for your health is not a shortcut, and it is not something you need to justify. It is an investment in your future.

As a Registered Dietitian with over 13 years expereince, I have had the privilege of working closely with many women navigating weight loss with the support of GLP-1 medications. I've celebrated their wins, helped them through their frustrations, and guided them past the confusion that often comes with dramatic appetite changes. What I've leared is this: the medication is a powerful tool, but it is not the whole strategy.

Introduction

Too many women are told to "eat less" and watch the scale drop. But rapid weight loss without the right nutriton and strength habits can cost you muscle, energy, metabolic health, and long-term success. My goal in writing this book is to make sure that doesn't happen to you.

This guide was created to help you lose fat in a way that supports your body rather than depletes it. Inside, you'll learn how to nourish yourself even when you're not hungry, protect your muscle, manage common side effects, and build habits that allow you to maintain your results - whether you stay on GLP-1 long term or eventually transition off.

You will not find shame, extremes, or rigid rules. Instead, you'll find evidence-based guidance, practical strategies, and a compassionate approach designed specifically for women.

I also want you to remember this: progress is not only measured by the number on the scale. It shows up in your strength, your confidence, your energy, and your ability to live your life more fully.

Whever you are starting from, you are not behind - and you are not alone.

Let's begin.

Health is not a moment in time but a journey with ebbs and flows. Prioritizing the journey is key.

Disclaimer

The information provided in this book is for educational and informational purposes only and is not intended as medical advice.

This content is not a substitute for professional medical evaluation, diagnosis, or treatment. Always seek the advice of your physician or other qualified healthcare provider with any questions you may have regarding a medical condition, medication, nutrition plan, or exercise program.

GLP-1 receptor agonists, including medications such as Ozempic, Wegovy, Mounjaro, and Zepbound, are prescription medications that must be prescribed and monitored by a licensed healthcare provider. Medication decisions, including initiation, dosing, tapering, or discontinuation, should always be made in consultation with your prescribing clinician.

The nutritional strategies, protein recommendations, strength training guidance, and behavioral frameworks discussed in this book are general in nature and may not be appropriate for every individual. Individual medical history, metabolic health, medications, injuries, lifestyle factors must be considered before implementing any changes.

The author makes no guarantees regarding specific outcomes. Results vary based on individual adherence, physiology, and health status.

If you experience adverse symptoms including severe abdominal pain, persistent vomiting, dehydration, dizziness, chest pain, or other concerning reactions while taking medication or beginning any new health regimen, seek immediate medical attention.

By reading this book, you acknowledge that you are responsible for your own health decisions and that the author and publisher are not liable for any injury, loss, or damages resulting from the application of the information provided.

Health is individual. Medical care is personal. Use this information as education - not prescription.

About Me

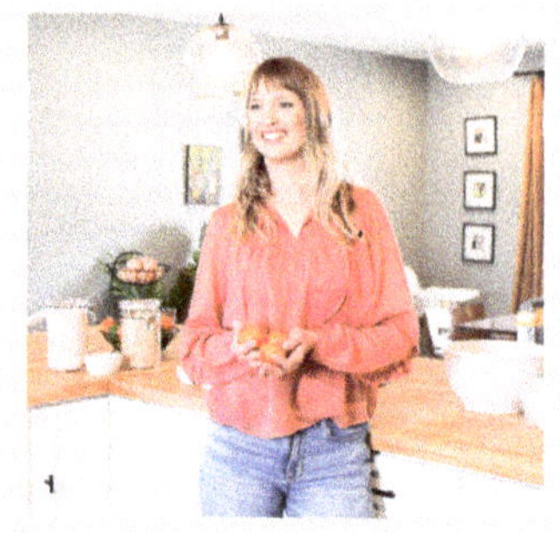

I grew up in the Blue Ridge Mountains in Virginia and earned by B.S. in Business Administration from Mary Washington University. After college, I discovered my love of wellness and became a Registered Dietitian with James Madison University and VCU Health Systems. I have over 13 years experience in clinical nutrition.

Even with my degree and training, I get it. Prioritizing health and making change stick is hard.

As a woman entering my 40s with two young kids, I have also struggled with my weight, nutrition, and body image over the years. Knowing what we *should* do is one thing...actually doing it while balancing a career, family, and any semblance of a social life is something else entirely.

On top of that, there is constant information coming at us from social media platforms, news, and influencers on what to do and what not to do to be healthier and lose weight. It's overwhelming.

That is why I have worked to cut through the noise for myself and now for you. This becomes even more important when on a GLP-1, when having clarity and a sustainable approach to health really matters.

You don't need to overhaul your life. You need a framework that works *within* it.

Anna, RD

Contents

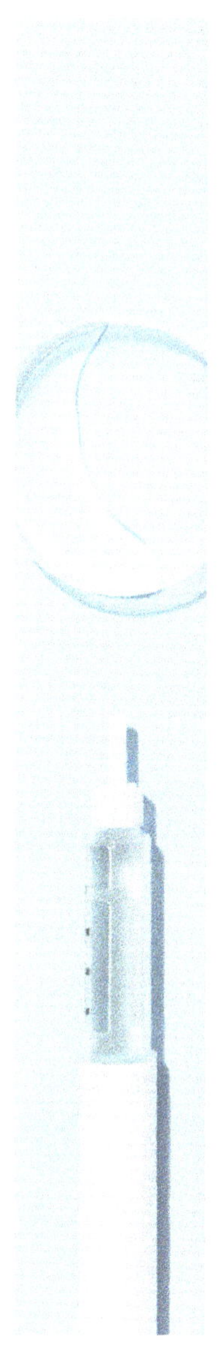

01 The Truth About GLP-1 Medications

GLP-1 Medications have changed the landscape of weight loss, especially for women who have spent years doing "everything right" and still struggle to see results.

For many, these medications feel like the first time their body is finally cooperating.

But with that relief comes confusion.

Are they safe long term?
Are you losing the right kind of weight?
What happens when you stop?
Is appetite suppression enough?

Let's clear the noise and talk about what's actually happening in your body.

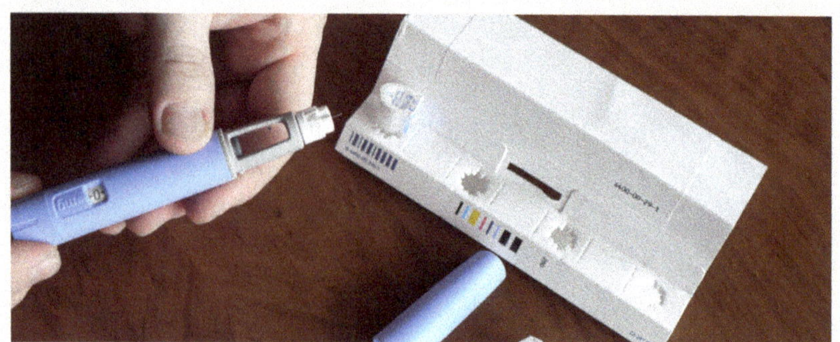

What is a GLP-1 Medication?

GLP-1 stands for glucagon-like peptide-1, a hormone your body naturally produces in the gut. It plays several roles in glucose and appetite regulation.[10]

Medications like semaglutide and tirzepatide mimic or enhance this hormone's effects in the body. [11, 34]

The result?

You feel full sooner.
You stay full longer.
Food noise quiets.

And that can feel life changing.

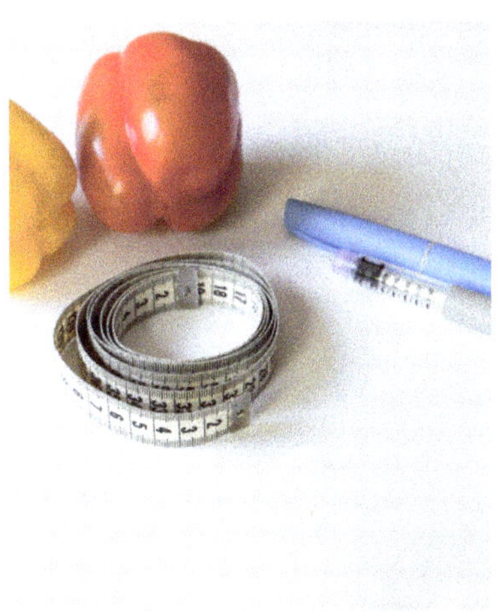

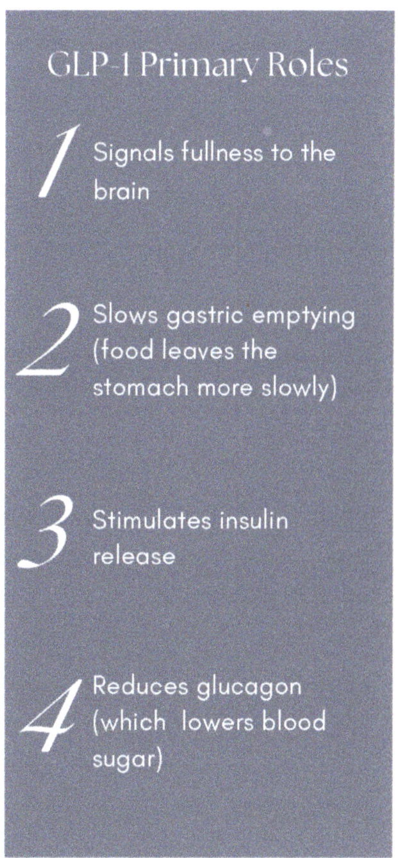

What GLP-1s Actually Do (And What They Don't)

There's a common misconception that these medications "boost metabolism."

They don't.

They primarily reduce caloric intake by reducing appetite and slowing digestion.

Weight loss happens because you are eating less – often significantly less.[4] This is constant with all diets; weight loss occurs due to a reduction of calories.

That clarification matters. Because while fat loss is the goal...your body doesn't only burn fat when calories drop.

It can also break down muscle.

The Hidden Risk: Muscle Loss

Rapid weight loss – especially when protein intake is low – increases the risk of losing lean muscle mass. This is not unique to GLP-1 medications, it occurs with most forms of significant weight loss.

Muscle is not just aesthetic though. Lean muscle:

- Protects your metabolic rate
- Supports blood sugar regulation
- Preserves strength and bone density
- Impacts how "tight" or "toned" your body looks

Research shows that up to 25-40% of weight loss without resistance training can come from lean mass.[34]

This is why some women feel:
- Softer instead of firmer
- More fatigued
- Colder
- Skinny but not strong[19]

The medication isn't the problem.

Lack of strategy is.

Appetite Suppression is a Tool - Not a Plan

One of the most common patterns I see in my practice: a women starts a GLP-1 medication, feels incredible appetite control, and begins eating very small amounts - sometimes unintentionally dropping below 1,000 calories a day.

At first, the scale drops quickly which can lead to empowerment and excitement.

But over time:
- Energy drops
- Hair may thin
- Workouts feel harder
- Plateaus appear
- Muscle loss increases

The body adapts to low intake.

GLP-1 medications reduce hunger signals. They do not replace your body's nutritional needs.

Why Some People Regain Weight

When someone stops a GLP-1 without building supportive habits, appetite often returns before structure does.[35]

If muscle mass was lost during rapid weight loss, metabolic rate may be lower than when they started.[32]

If appetite returns and muscle mass was not preserved, the environment becomes primed for regain. It turns into the viscious cycle of yo-yo dieting that many of us are all too familiar with.

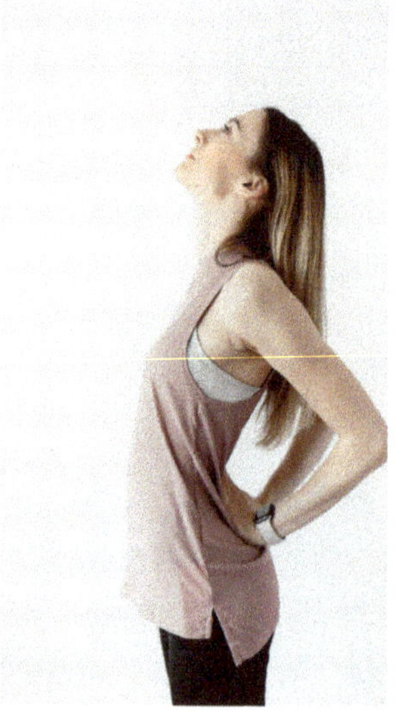

Regain is more likely without:

- Adequate protein
- Strength training
- High fiber intake
- Lifestyle rhythm promoting stress relief

GLP-1 helps manage appetite. It does not teach sustainable eating habits.

That is what this book is for.

The Opportunity

When used strategically, GLP-1 medications create a unique opportunity to:

- Reduce food noise
- Improve insulin sensitivity
- Improve control around eating to set better habits[11]

Instead of white-knuckling hunger, you can focus on building habits.

This is an ideal time to:

- Prioritize protein
- Build strength
- Establish meal rhthym
- Improve sleep and stress patterns

This is not about eating less.

It's about eating intentionally.

Before moving forward, let's take 5 minutes to reflect...

Your Starting Point

1. What has weight loss felt like for me in the past?

2. What am I most afraid of while taking GLP-1?

3. Do I want fast weight loss - or sustainable body change?

4. Am I currently strength training? If not, why?

5. How much protein am I eating most days?
   You can estimate this using any calorie counting app to track protein.

The #1 Mistake People Make on GLP-1

02

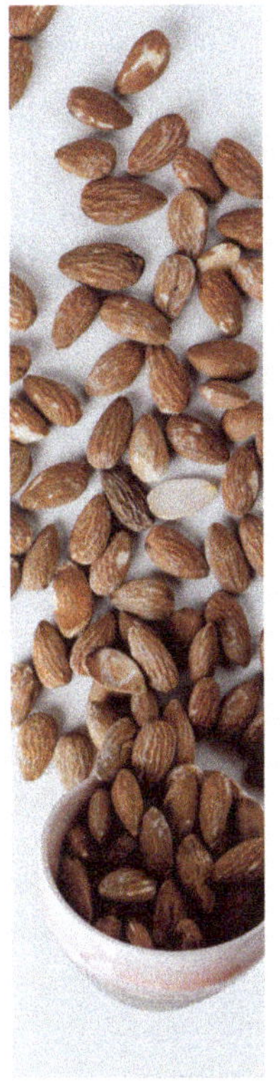

> *Protecting muscle while you lose fat is the key to long term success.*

If GLP-1 medications reduce appetite, protein preserves metabolism.

This is the strategy most people are not taught and the one that determines whether weight loss leaves you feeling strong or depleted.

Most people assume eating less will set them up for success but this will just set you up for yo-yo weight changes.

Why Protein Matters More on a GLP-1

When calorie intake drops, the body does not selectively burn fat. Let's say that again for those in the back - when calorie intake drops, the body does NOT just go into 'fat burning' mode.

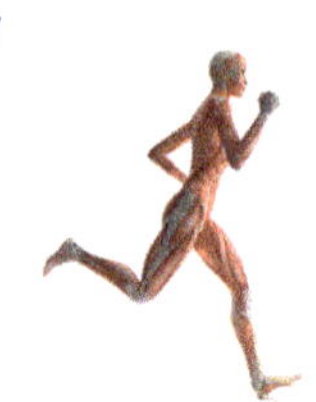

It uses both fat mass and lean mass for energy.[32]

Lean Mass Includes:

- Skeletal muscle
- Organs
- Connective tissue
- Water assosciated with muscle

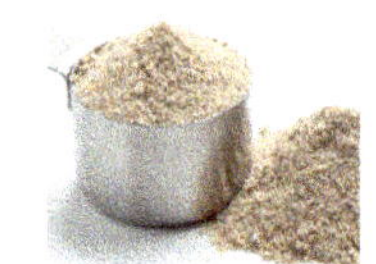

Muscle is metabolically active tissue. It plays a centrol role in:

- Glucose disposal
- Resting metabolic rate
- Strength and function
- Long-term weight maintenance[37]

Higher protein intake during weight loss has been shown to:

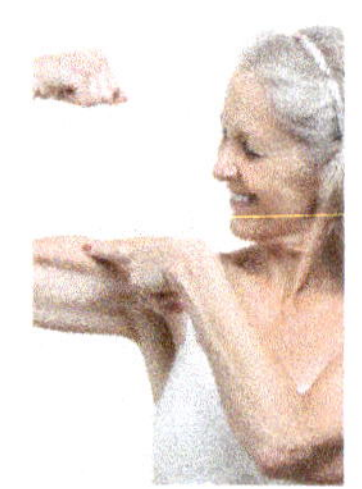

- Reduce loss of lean body mass
- Improve feeling of fullness (satiety)
- Support fat loss while preserving muscle[12, 22]

For women on GLP-1 medications - who may intentionally eat very little - higher protein intake becomes non-negotiable.

How Much Protein Do You Actually Need?

The standard Recommended Dietary Allowance (RDA) for protein is 0.36 grams per pound body weight (often discussed as 0.8 g/kg).

This is the minimum required to prevent deficiency, *not the optimal amount for fat loss.*

During caloric restriction, research supports increasing protein intake to 0.6-0.7 grams per pound body weight per day.[22]

For individuals resistance training during weight loss (like you, right?) intakes toward the higher end may further preserve lean mass.[18]

A practical clinical recommendation:

0.7-1.0 grams protein per pound of goal body weight

This range supports muscle retention while remaining achievalbe even with appetite suppression.

Let's calculate your goal protein range.

Your goal weight: _____________ x 0.7 = lower range goal ___________
Your goal weight: _____________ x 1.0 = upper range goal ___________

Daily protein goal (lower - upper): _______________________ grams

Protein and Fullness

Protein has the highest satiety effect of all macronutrients.
It influences:

- Peptide YY
- GLP-1 secretion
- Ghrelin suppression

This means prioritizing protein works synergistically with your medication.[12]

Instead of relying solely on appetite suppression, you are reinforcing fullness through physiology.

The Muscle Preservation Formula

To protect muscle while losing fat on a GLP-1:

1. Eat sufficient protein daily (in the range you just calculated based on your goal weight)
2. Distribute protein evenly across meals
3. Incoprorate resistance training

Protein Distribution Matters

Research shows that distributing protein evenly across meals (approximately 25-40 grams per meal) improves muscle protein synthesis compared to skewing intake towards dinner.[16]

Because appetite is often lowest later in the day on GLP-1 medications, intentional planning is necessary.

Even small meals should anchor around protein.

Practical Protein Strategies When You Are Not Hungry

Appetite suppression can make large meals uncomfortable. Use these strategies...

1. Protein First - take 5 to 10 bites of protein before anything else
2. Think Smaller, Not Less - instead of 3 large meals consider 4 small protein focused meals or 3 meals and 1 to 2 protein snacks
3. Use Liquid Nutrition Strategically - protein smoothies or greek yogurt can be easier to tolerate when fullness is high
4. Keep It Simple
   a. Greek yogurt + berries
   b. Cottage cheese + fruit
   c. Eggs + avocado
   d. Chicken + roasted veggies
   e. Oatmeal + protein powder

Remember chronic under-eating:

- Increases lean mass loss
- Reduces resting energy expenditure
- Increases fatigue
- Slows metabolic rates through adaptive thermogenesis[19]

The goal is not just weight loss. The goal is fat loss.

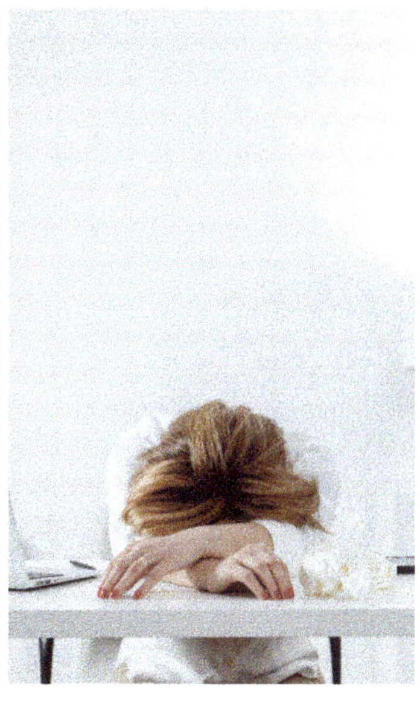

Self - Assessment Checklist

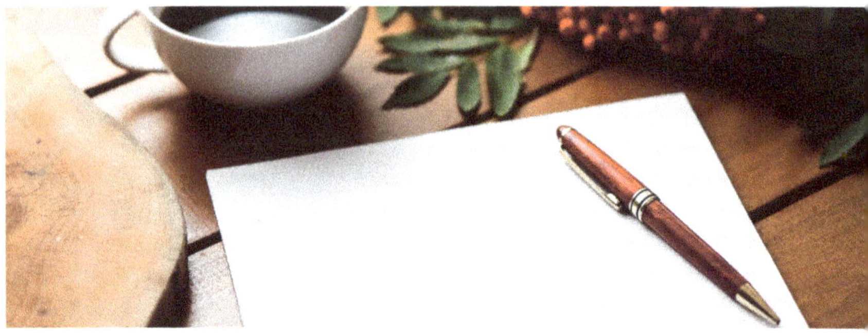

<table>
<tr><td>Step 1 Calculate Target Protein</td><td>Goal weight:_____________________

Protein range (0.7-1.0 g/lb):_____g/day</td></tr>
<tr><td>Step 2 Divide Your Meals</td><td>Goal protein _____ grams Divided by meals/per day

Meal 1:_______________________
Meal 2:_______________________
Meal 3:_______________________
Meal 4 or snacks:________________</td></tr>
<tr><td>Self Assessment Checklist</td><td>✓ I know my protein target

✓ I include protein at every meal

✓ I resistance train at least 2-3 times per week

✓ I am not constantly eating below 1,200 calories</td></tr>
</table>

Protein Powder Comparison

Protein powders can be a strategic tool, especially when appetite is low and you need to maximize calories but not all protein powders are created equal.

Type	Best For	Benefits	Things to Consider	When to Use	What to Look For
Whey Protein Isolate	Most people	Fast absorption, high leucine, excellent for muscle preservation	Contains small amounts of lactose (usually tolerated well)	Post-workout	>20 g protein, < 3g sugar per scoop; third party tested[28]
Whey Protein Concen trate	Budget-friendly option	Contains beneficial bioactive compounds, creamy texture	Slightly more lactose	Smoothies or meal replacement	>20 g protein, < 3g sugar per scoop; third party tested[7]
Casein Protein	Evening use	Slow-digesting; promotes fullness; sustsained amino acid release	Thicker texture	Before bed, long gaps between meals	> 20 g protein; minimal fillers[5]
Pea Protein	Dairy-Free vegan option	Good amino acid profile; hypoallergenic	Slightly lower leucine than whey	Smoothies; plant based diets	Blended with rice protein for completeness[2]
Soy Protein	Plant-based complete protein	Contains all amino acids	Some avoid due to personal preference	Meal replacement smoothies	Non-GMO preferred[17]
Collage n Peptide s	Skin/joint support	Supports connective tissue	Not a complete protein; low leucine	Add to yogurt, coffee	Use as supplement – not replacement for protein[25]
Protein Blends	Balanced digestion speed	Ccmbines fast and slow proteins	Quality varies widely	Anytime protein boost	Transparent ingredient list

Understanding Leucine & Why It Matters

Leucine is the key amino acid that stimulates muscle protein synthesis.[28]

Research suggests that about 2-3 grams leucine per meal optimally stimulates muscle repair and preservation.[20]

Whey isolate is particularly effective because of its high leucine concentration.[28]

This matters on GLP-1 medications where total intake may be lower and preserving lean mass is critical.[32]

When to Use Protein Powder Strategically

Protein powder is helpful when:
- Breakfast protein intake is low
- Appetite is supressed
- Post-workout intake is delayed
- Travel disrupts routine
- Daily protein intake is below 100 g

It is a supplement - not a replacement for whole food.

Avoid protein powders with a long artificial ingredient list, 6-8+ grams added sugars, "proprietary blends" without transparency, excessive "proprietary fat burners," and unverified health claims.

Look for:
- Third party testing (NSF, Informed Sport, or USP)
- Clear protein amount per serving
- Simple ingredient list

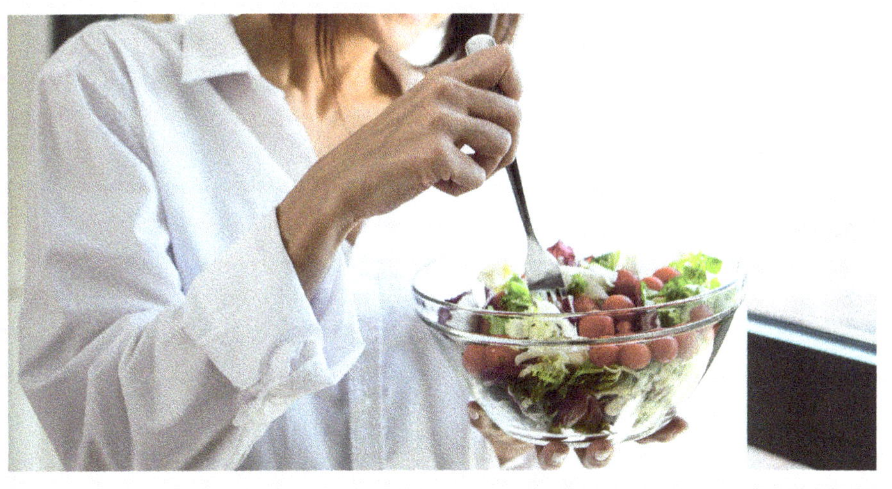

03

How to Eat When You're Not Hungry

The key to sustainable weight loss is ensuring habits are sustainable as well.

How to Eat When You Aren't Hungry

One of the most common things I hear from women on GLP-1 medications is:

"I'm just not hungry anymore. I'm just not eating that much."

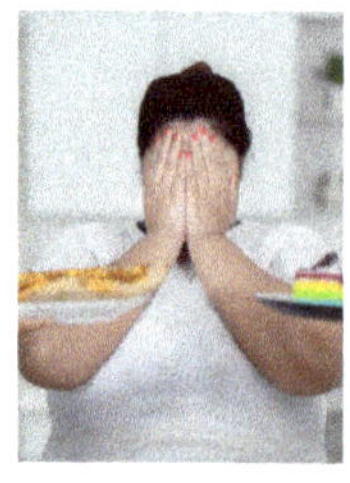

For many, this feels like relief after years of constant food noise.

But appetite suppression can create a new problem:

You still need nourishment - even when hunger is quiet.

Why Hunger Changes on GLP-1 Medications

GLP-1 receptor agonists act on appetite-regulating centers in the brain, including the hypothalamus, and influence satiety hormones such as peptide YY while reducing ghrelin, the hunger hormone.[4]

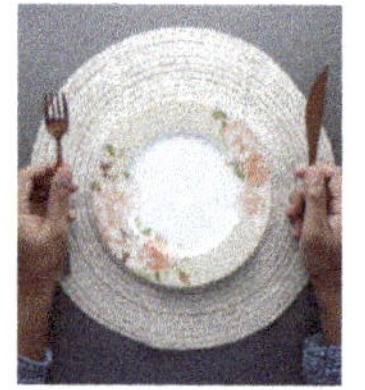

GLP-1's also slow gastric emptying, meaning food stays in the stomach longer.[10]

Fullness does not eliminate your body's need for:

- Protein
- Essential fatty acids
- Micronutrients
- Adequate total energy

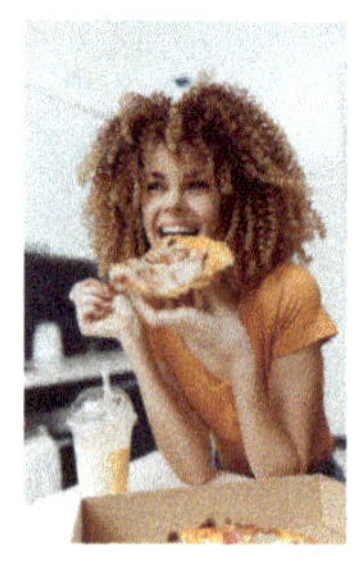

When intake drops too low for too long, the body adapts and your results will slow if not reverse.[19]

The GLP-1 Eating Framework

When appetite is low, shift from "How much can I eat?" to:
"What is the most nutritionally effiecient way to eat?"

Step 1 - Prioritize Protein First

Protein supports muscle protein synthesis, especially during caloric restriction so you will retain lean muscle.[18]

When you sit down to eat: Start with protein.

Even 15-25 grams of protein is meaningful if appetite is low.

Examples:
- ¾ cup greek yogurt
- 2 eggs with 2 egg whites
- 3-4 oz of chicken
- Protein smoothie

The Risk of Chronically Eating Too Little

- ✔ Increased lean muscle mass loss[32]
- ✔ Reduced resting energy expenditure[19]
- ✔ Micronutrient deficiencies, such as B12, vitamin D, magnesium
- ✔ Fatgue and impaired training recovery
- ✔ Increased hair loss

Step 2 - Think Small, Not Sparse

Instead of large meals, try 4 smaller meals or 3 small meals and 1-2 snacks.

Large portions may feel overwhelming due to delayed gastric emptying.

Smaller meals can:
- Improve food tolerance
- Reduce nausea
- Support more consistent intake

Step 3 - Use Liquid Nutrition Strategically

Liquids empty from the stomach more easily than solid food.

This makes protein smoothies or drinkable yogurt useful tools when fullness is high. Protein shakes can also be a great way to get high amounts of protein in without meat.

Example smoothie structure:
- 1 scoop protein powder
- 1 cup Greek yogurt of milk
- 1 Tbsp nut butter or chia seeds
- 1/2-1 cup frozen berries
- 1 cup spinach

I typically only recommend protein powders/liquid nutrition no more than once a day. As always, I prefer real food first as powders can have additional sugars, additives, and potential for heavy metals.

Step 4 - Avoid the "Only Carbs" Trap

When appetite is low, it's common to reach for carbohydrate foods such as toast, crackers, fruit, chips, and other snack foods.

These are easy to tolerate but low in protein and potentially low in micronutrients.

Carbohydrates are a great energy source for the body but they alone do not sufficiently stimulate muscle protein synthesis.[18]

Always anchor carbohydrates to protein.

For example: instead of just toast. Try:
- Eggs + toast
- Cottage cheese + toast
- Greek yogurt + toast

Step 5 - Manage Nausea Without Sacraficing Nutrition

If nausea occurs:
- Eat slowly
- Choose bland but protein rich foods
- Avoid high-fat meals initially
- Stay hydrated

Persistent nausea should be discussed with your healthcare provider.

A Note on Intermitten Fasting

Intermittent fasting (IF) is often discussed alongside weight loss.
But it is important to understand what it is, and what it is not.

Intermittent fasting is not a specific diet but a timing strategy.

Common approaches include:
- 16:8 – 16 hours fasting and 8 hour eating window
- 14:10 – 14 hours fasting and 10 hour eating window
- Alternate day fasting
- 24 hour fasts 1-2 times per week

The question is not whether intermittent fasting 'works' but the better question is does it work for you? Especially when using a GLP-1 medication.

What Research Shows

Studies suggest intermittent fasting can:
- Reduce total calorie intake
- Improve insulin sensitivity
- Support weight loss comprable to traditional calorie restriction
- Improve certain cardiometabolic markers[9]

Research shows that weight loss results from overall calorie reduction, not from fasting as a metabolic boost.[14]

For women specifically moderate time-restricted eating (especially a 12-14 overnight fast) is safe and sustainable.[36]
However for women, more aggressive fasting protocols may increase stress hormones, especially in women who are already under-eating.[6]

A Note on Intermitten Fasting

When appetite is suppressed from GLP-1 medications, some women unintentionally skip breakfast, eat one or two small meals, and therefore struggle to meet daily protein requirements.

While this may accelerate scale weight loss initially, it can increase risk of lean mass loss, fatigue, and slower metabolic adaptations over time.[34]

If you are already eating less because of the medication, layering aggressive fasting on top may not be beneficial.

When Intermittent Fasting May Be Helpful:

Intermittent Fasting may be useful if:

- It simplifies your routine
- It reduces mindless snacking, especially at night
- You can still hit protein targets
- Energy levels remain stable
- Strength training performance is preserved[27]

When Intermittent Fasting May Backfire:

Consider adjusting or avoiding fasting if:

- Difficulty meeting protein goals
- Increased dizziness or nausea
- Low energy during workouts
- Hair thinning
- Heightened stress/irritability
- Loss of menstrual regularity[15]

For women, chronic under-fueling can disrupt hormonal balance. The goal is metabolic support, not additional stress.

Hydration & Electrolytes

Reduced food intake often means reduced sodium intake.

Symptoms of low sodium or dehydration include:

- Headaches
- Fatigue
- Dizziness
- Weakness

Adequate hydration supports digestion and overall well-being.[26]

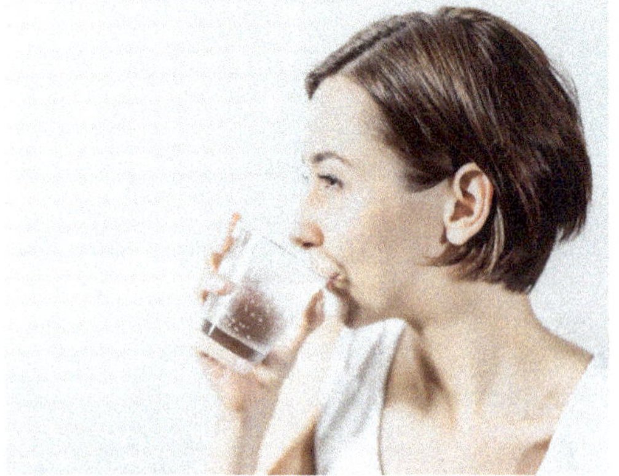

While individual needs vary, most adults benefit from consistent fluid intake throughout the day.

You shouldn't need specific electrolyte replacement unless you are sweating heavily or working out longer than an hour a day.

Electrolyte Replacement: Evidence, Options & Practical Use

Electrolytes regulate fluid balance, neuromuscular signaling, and blood pressure. Sodium in particular plays a critical role in plasma volume and orthostatic stability.[26]

Low-carbohydrate intake and fasting reduce circulating insulin, which increases renal sodium excretion.[8] This is why women following GLP-1 medicaitons combined with lower food intake may experience headaches, fatigue, dizziness upon standing, and muscle cramps.

Exercise-related sweat losses can further increase sodium requirements, particularly in warm climates.[1]

When to Use Electrolytes

Step 1. Are you experiencing any of the following?
- Lightheadedness when standing
- Persistent headaches
- Muscle cramps
- Rapid fatigue during workouts
- Dark Urine
- Salt cravings

If NO
Focus on consistent water intake first.

If YES
Continue to Step 2.

When to Use Electrolytes

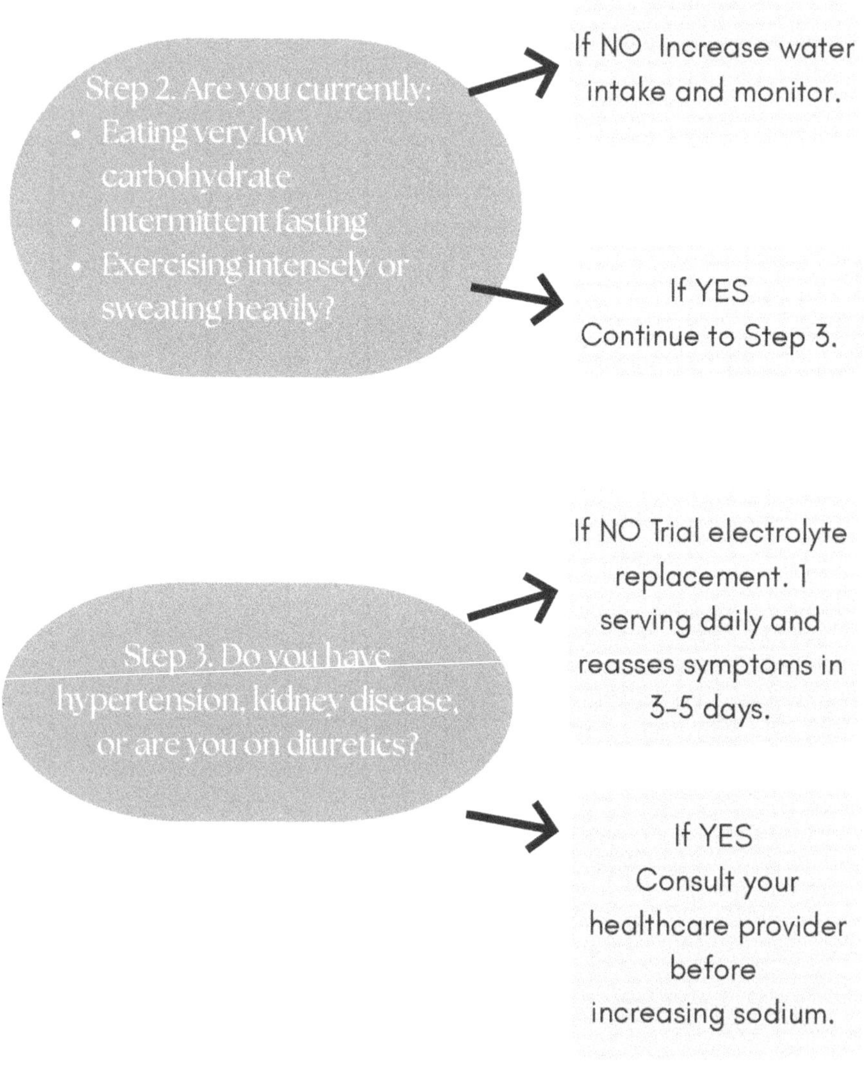
Step 2. Are you currently:
Eating very low carbohydrate
Intermittent fasting
Exercising intensely or sweating heavily?
If NO Increase water intake and monitor.
If YES Continue to Step 3.
Step 3. Do you have hypertension, kidney disease, or are you on diuretics?
If NO Trial electrolyte replacement. 1 serving daily and reasses symptoms in 3-5 days.
If YES Consult your healthcare provider before increasing sodium.

Electrolyte Comparison Chart

Product	Sodium (approx)	Potassium	Magnesium	Sugar	Best For	Notes
LMNT	1000 mg	200 mg	60 mg	0 g	Low-carb, heavy sweaters	High sodium, no sugar
Liquid I.V.	500 mg	370 mg	Trace amt	11 g	Exercise, mild dehydration	Contains glucose for absorption
Nuun Sport	300 mg	150 mg	25 mg	1 g	Light workouts	Convenient tablet form
Ultima Replenisher	55 mg	250 mg	100 mg	0 g	Daily light hydration	Lower sodium option

Please check labels on electrolyte replacement for current product specifications and accurate levels.

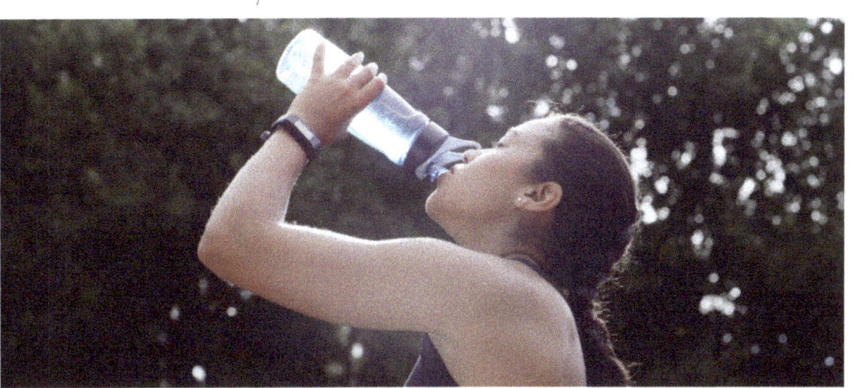

Your Low-Appetite Plan

1. When is my appetite highest during the day?

2. When is my appetite the lowest during the day?

3. Which protein foods feel easiest to eat?

4. What is one liquid protein option I can keep available?

5. Am I intentionally skipping meals? Does this seem to affect my hunger and energy later in the day?

04 Strength Training: The Muscle Preservation Plan

If protein protects muscle nutritionally, strength training protects it mechanically.

When losing weight - especially quickly - resistance training is NOT optional.

It is protective medicine.

Why Muscle Matters More Than the Scale?

Most women starting a GLP-1 want to see the scale move. And it likely will.
But the scale does not distinguish between fat mass, lean mass, and water.

During caloric restriction, lean mass loss can account for 20-40% of total weight lost if no resistance training is performed.[32]

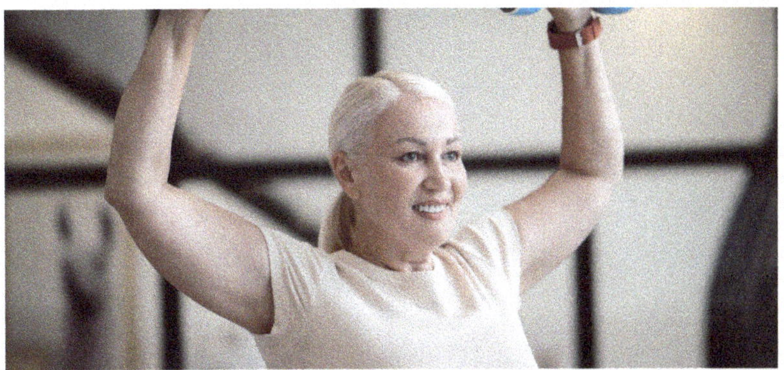

Are You At Risk of "Soft" Weight loss?

GLP-1 medications reduce appetite and total energy intake.[4]

Without mechanical stimulus (strength training), the body adapts to lower intake by reducing energy expenditure and breaking down lean tissue.[19]

This can lead to reduced strength, lower resting metabolic weight, "skinny-fat" appearance, and increased fatigue.

Weight loss without muscle preservation changes body composition in ways that are not always visible on the scale - but are very real physiologically.

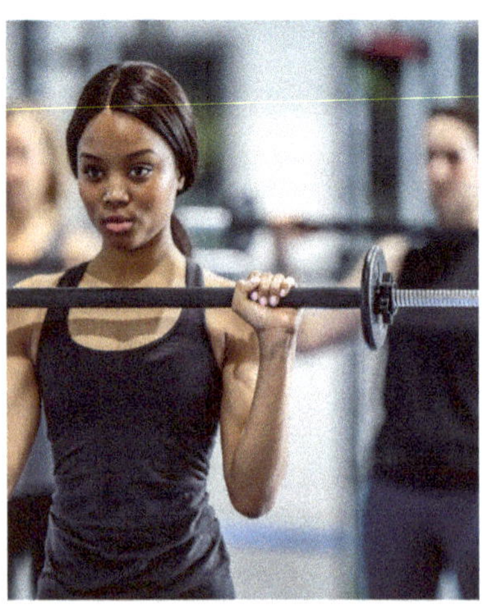

Benefits of Skeletal Muscle

1 Regulates glucose disposal

2 Supports resting metabolic rate

3 Protects bone density

4 Reduces fall risk

5 Improves long term weight maintenance[37]

The Metabolism Connection

Resting metabolic rate (RMR) accounts for the majority of energy expenditure. So unless you are running marathons, most of your calorie 'burn' comes from day to day activity like breathing, thinking, walking, digesting food, etc.

Lean mass is one of the strongest predictors of RMR (not weight!).[37]

During weight loss, RMR declines due to reduced body mass. Adaptive thermogenesis may further suppress energy expenditure.[19]

While some metabolic adaptation is expected, maintaining lean mass reduces the degree of slowdown of your RMR.

This becomes especially important if medication is discontinued.

Strength Training and Aging

For women, especially over 35-40, preserving muscle is also about aging well.

Resistance training:
- Improves bone mineral density
- Reduces sarcopenia risk (progressive muscle loss after 30)
- Improves insulin sensitivity
- Enhances functional capacity[33]

Rapid weight loss without strength training may accelerate visible and functional signs of aging as muscles give structure to the body and face.

If you have not made strength training a part of your weekly routine yet, this is your sign to start. It's not too late.

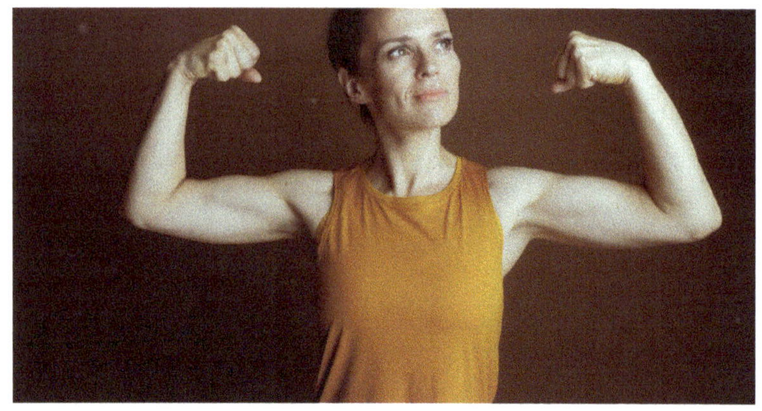

What Counts as Strength Training?

Exercises like light pilates (without progression) and yoga are very beneficial and are a great way to improve your health. However, they do not provide enough stimulus to preserve muscle during weight loss and would not count towards your weekly strength training plan.

Strength training means progressive overload applied to muscle:

- Free weights
- Machine weights
- Resistance bands
- Body weight movements (if challenging enough)

It does NOT include:
- Light Pilates
- Casual yoga
- Walking

I often hear "I don't need the gym. I am on my feet all day." Unfortunately that is NOT ENOUGH. You must be adding in true resistance training!

The GLP-1 Strength Blueprint

Minimum Effective Structure

Frequency: 2-4 sessions per week

Duration: 30-45 minutes

Focus: Compound Movements

Include upper and lower body lifting along with core work.

Squats	Rows	Bicep Curls
Deadlifts	Chest press/push ups	Tricep extensions
Lunges	Shoulder press	Planks

What if Energy is Low?

Fatigue can occur early during GLP-1 titration.

If energy is reduced:

- Shorten sessions of strength training
- Reduce volume, not intensity
- Prioritize compound lifts
- Ensure protein and hydration intake is adequate

Even one focused session a week is better than none.

What About Cardio?

Cardio has cardiovascular benefits but during calorie restriction, excessive cardio without resistance training can increase muscle loss.[32]

Always strength train first if time is limited.

Consider adding in daily walks or light cardio a few times a week if energy and time permits.

Your Strength Commitment

Please consult with a doctor or medical provider before starting a new exercise program.

1. Am I currently strength training consistently?

2. If not, what are the real barriers?

3. How many days per week can I realistically commit?

4. Do I need guidance like a trainer, program, class, or app? If so, what will I use?

(Popular choices include Peloton app, Stronger by the Day app, Fitness Blender)

5. What time of day works best for me?

Your Strength Commitment

I commit to strengh training _________
days a week for the next 8 weeks.

I am going to use the following
program to strength train

____.

The days I am aiming to work out on
are____

____

____.

The time of day I am going to work out
during is _______________________________.

I will fuel my body before and after by

____

____.

05 Managing Side Effects: A Practical Nutrition-First Approach

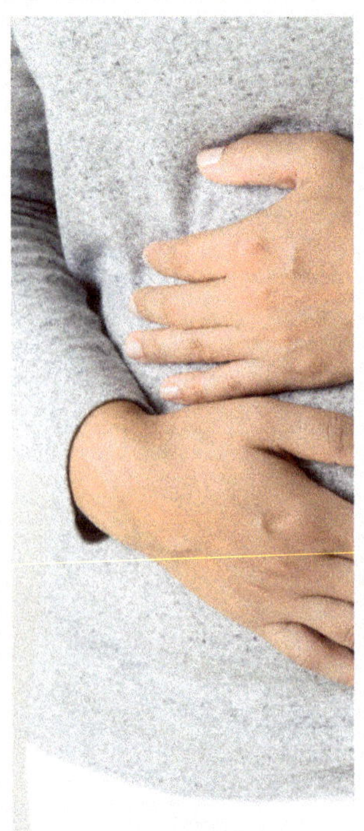

GLP-1 medications are highly effective but like all medications they are not side-effect free.

Most side effects are gastrointestinal and dose-dependent. They often occur during escalation and improve over time.[34]

The key is not the power through discomfort.

It's to adjust strategically.

This chapter will help you understand what is happening physiologically and how to respond to manage these side effects.

Why Side Effects Happen

As discussed, GLP-1 receptor agonists slow gastric emptying, increase fullness signaling, alter the gut-brain communication, and influence insulin and glucagon secretion.[10]

The slowed gastric emptying is the primary driver of many symptoms.

Food sits in the stomach longer. For some, this produces therapeutic fullness.

For others it produces nausea, bloating, early satiety, and reflux.

If already experiences reflux and other GI symptoms prior to starting GLP-1, they are more likely to have these problems exacerbated.

Food choices can make these side effects worse, or better.

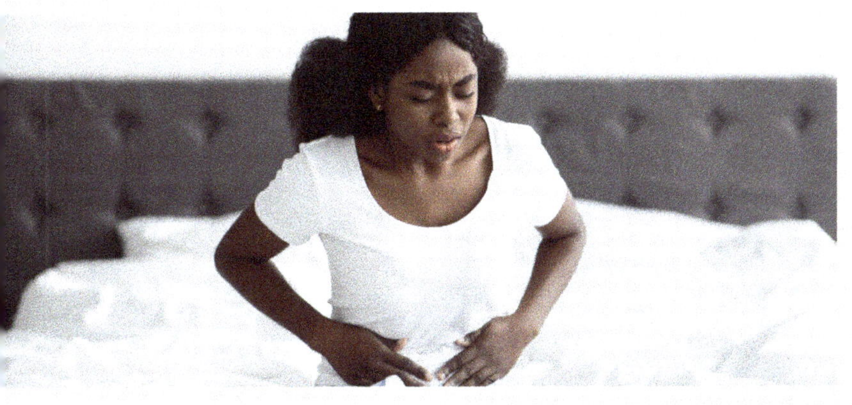

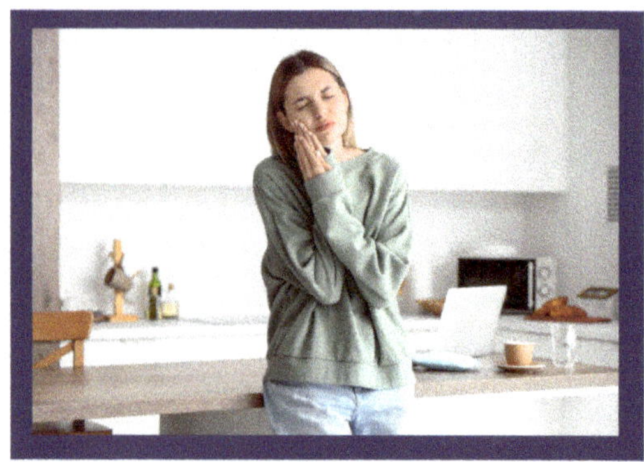

Nausea

Why it happens?

Delayed gastric emptying and central appetite regulation changes can increase nausea, especially during dose increases.[34]

Nutrition Strategies

1. Eat slowly
2. Stop at comfortable fullness, not stuffed
3. Avoid large, high-fat meals which delays gastric emptying further
4. Choose smaller, protein-forward meals
5. Avoid lying down immediately after eating
6. Try ginger tea or ginger chews

When to Call Your Provider

- Persistent vomiting
- Inability to keep fluids down
- Signs of dehydration (reduced urination, fatigue, dry mouth, dizziness, headaches)

Constipation

Why it happens?

Reduced food intake, particularly reduced fiber intake, slowed GI motility, and lower fluid intake all contribute to constipation.

Prevention Strategies

1. Fiber

Aim for 21-30 grams of fiber per day. Increase your fiber gradually to avoid worsening bloating.

2. Fluids

Aim to drink at least 2-2.5 liters of water per day unless medically contraindicated.

3. Movement

Daily walking and exercise helps stimulate bowl movements.

Helpful Foods

- Chia seeds (add to protein smoothies or yogurt)
- Ground flax
- Certain fruits – kiwi, pears, apples with skin
- Oats
- Lentils and other beans
- Vegetables

If needed discuss a magnesium or stool softener with your provider. I encourage you to focus on the 3 prevention strategies first.

Fatigue

Why it happens?

Possible causes include reduced calorie intake, low protein intake, dehydration, low sodium intake, and rapid weight loss.

Practical Fixes

- Ensure adequate protein intake
- Avoid chronically eating under 1,200 calories per day without supervision
- Add electrolytes to your water if experiencing dizziness or headaches
- Prioritize sleep

Hair Shedding

Hair thinning is distressing but not uncommon during rapid weight loss.

Why is happens?

Telogen effluvium is a temporary condition where the body's stress response forces hair follicles into a resting phase due to nutrient deficiencies.[22]

Prevention Strategies

- Maintain adequate protein intake
- Avoid extreme calorie restriction
- Ensure iron, zinc, and overall micronutrient adequacy
- Slow the rate of weight loss, if excessive

Why it happens?

Because gastric emptying is slowed, reflux symptoms may increase especially if prone to this prior to GLP-1.

Prevention Strategies

- Smaller meals
- Avoid eating within 2-3 hours of bed
- Limit high-fat meals, especially at night
- Sit upright after eating

If symptoms persist, consult your provider.

Muscle Loss

A sustainable weight loss of 1-3 pounds per week is ideal.

Consult with your provider if you are seeing larger jumps.

If weight is dropping quickly but strength is declining, lean mass may be decreasing.

Prevention Strategies

- Increase protein
- Add or increase resistance training
- Slow weight loss if needed

Remember, this is a marathon not a sprint and slower results can help preserve muscle mass and lead to more long term success in keeping your weight loss off!

Consider using a body composition machine regularly to look at your body fat and muscle percentage (versus just weight) to get a more accurate picture.

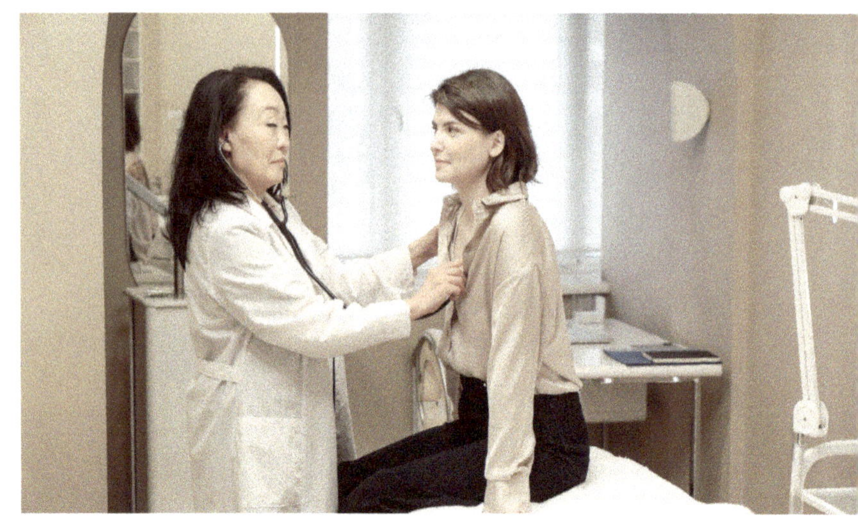

Red Flag Warning Symptoms

Most side effects are manaegable and are often dose-dependent, nutrition related, or adjustment related.

Strategic fueling, hydration, and muscle preservation dramatically reduce complications.

This medication creates the opportunity.

Your structure determines the experience.

Seek medical care for any of the following symptoms:

- Persistent severe abdominal pain
- Repeated vomiting
- Signs of pancreatitis (severe upper abdominal pain radiating to the back)
- Persistent dehydration
- Severe weakness

This book is educational and does not replace medical care.

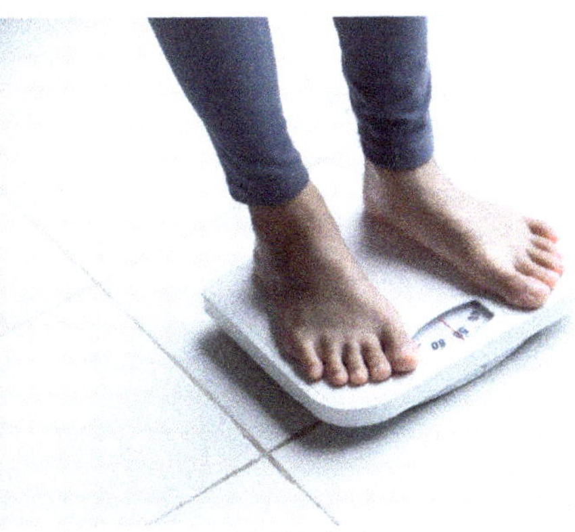

06

Body Composition, "Ozempic Face," and Why Rate of Loss Matters

You may have heard the phrase "Ozempic face." Its a media term, not a medical diagnosis, used to describe facial volume loss during rapid weight reduction. But here's the truth: It's not a medication-specific phenomenon, it is a rapid weight loss phenomenon. And understanding the difference matters.

What Actually Happens to Cause "Ozempic Face"?

When you lose weight you lose:
- Subcutaneous fat
- Visceral fat
- Water
- Glycogen
- Lean mass (if not protected)

Facial fullness is largely supported by:
- Subcutaneous fat (fat right under the skin)
- Skin elasticity
- Collagen structure

Rapid fat loss, especially without muscle preservation, can create:
- Hollowing under the eyes
- Cheek flattening
- Increased skin laxity
- More visible nasolabial folds

This is not unique to GLP-1 therapy. It can occur with bariatric surgery, very low calorie diets, and aggressive crash dieting.

The key variable is the speed of weight loss.[32]

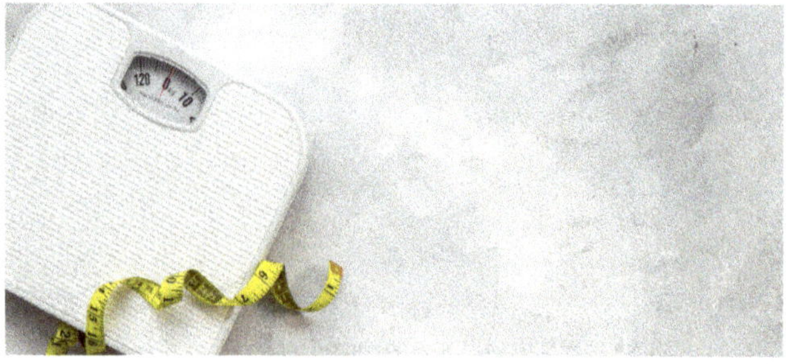

Collagen, Skin, & Aging

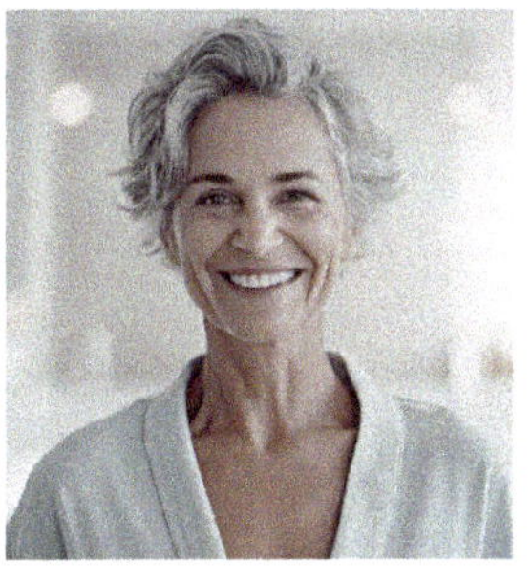

Skin elasticity declines naturally with age.

Rapid weight loss can unmask this decline.

While nutrition cannot fully prevent skin changes, it can support tissue integrity.
Key nutrients involved in collagen production:
- Protein (amino acids, especially glycine and proline)
- Vitamin C
- Zinc
- Copper

Severe calorie restriction may compromise micronutrient intake.
Adeqeuate protein during weight loss supports tissue presevation.[22]

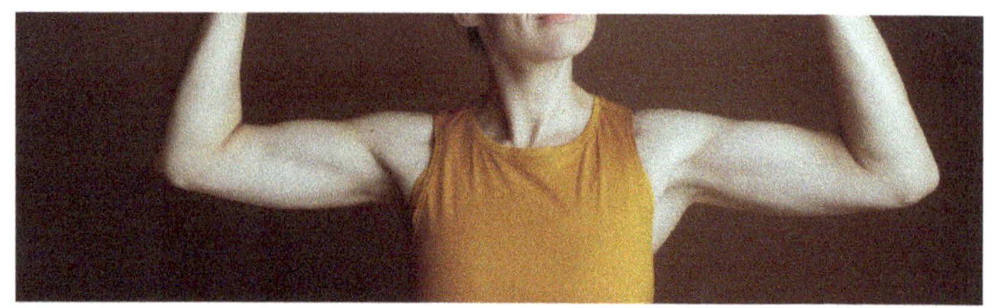

Protecting Body Composition on GLP-1

To minimize unwanted aesthetic and metabolic changes:

1. Prioritize Protein
Aim for 0.7-1.0 gram per pound body weight during caloric restriction.

2. Strength Train Consistently
2-4 Sessions per week minimum

The Psychological Component

Rapid changes in appearance can be emotionally disorienting. Even positive scale changes can feel unfamiliar. Some women report looking older, feeling less "filled out" and losing curves. This is why body composition matters more than body weight.

3. Avoid Extreme Caloric Restriction
Do not chronically under eat below 1,200 calories without medical supervision

4. Monitor Rate of Loss
If losing more than 2 pounds per week consistently, assess intake and muscle preservation strategy

5. Hydrate
Adequate hydration supports skin appearance and overall function.

Interactive Reflection

Fat Loss + Muscle Retention = Shape Change
Fat Loss + Muscle Loss = Shrinkage

1. How quickly am I currently losing weight?

2. Am I tracking strength improvements, or only the scale?

3. Do I feel stronger? Weaker? Unchanged?

4. Am I comfortable with my current rate of change?

5. What matters more to me - speed or body composition?

Reframing the Goal

Instead of asking: "How fast can I lose weight?"

Ask: "How well can I lose fat while preserving muscle?"

GLP-1 medications are powerful tools. But your strategy determines whether the result is smaller or stronger and leaner.

There are clinical cases, such as significant obesity with metabolic complications, where more rapid initial loss may be beneficial under supervision.

Even then muscle preservation strategies remain essential.

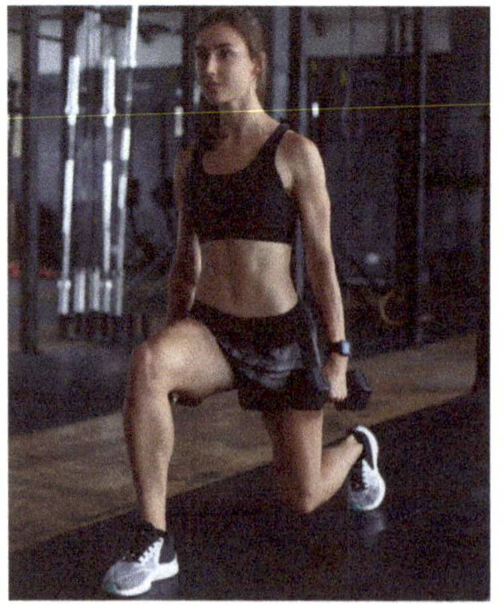

Clinical Takeaway

"Ozempic face" is not caused by the medication alone.

it is a reflection of:
- Rapid fat loss
- Lean mass lost
- Reduced structural support

With adequate protein, resistance training, and a controlled rate of loss, body composition outcomes dramatically improve.

The goal is not just less weight.

The goal is better composition.

07 When Weight Loss Stalls: Understanding Plateaus and Metabolic Adaption

At some point, the scale may stop moving even on ozempic.

Not for a day.
Not for a week.
But for several weeks.

This does not mean the medication has failed. It does not mean you are doing something wrong.
It does not mean that you need to eat less.

It means that your body is adapting.

And adaptation is normal physiology.

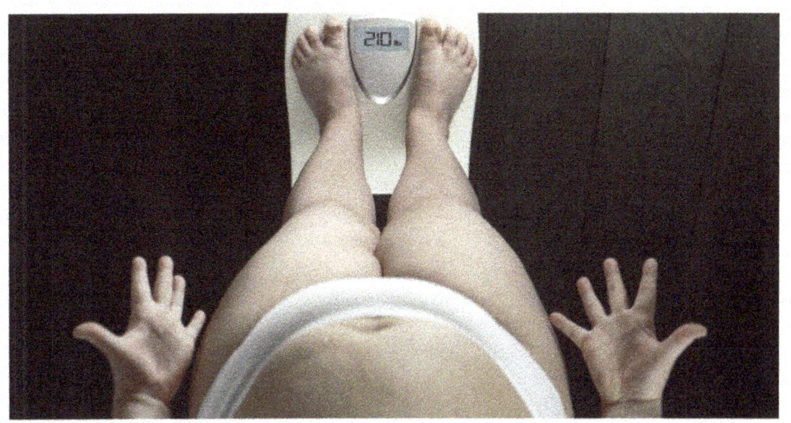

What is a True Plateau?

A true plaetau is no measurable weight change for 3-4 consecutive weeks while adherence to nutrition and movement remains consistent.

Short-term fluctuations are not pleasant but need to be expected.

Body weight naturally shifts due to :

- Glycogen changes
- Hydration
- Sodium intake
- Hormonal fluctuations
- Bowel patterns

Fat loss can occur even when scale weight temporarily stalls.

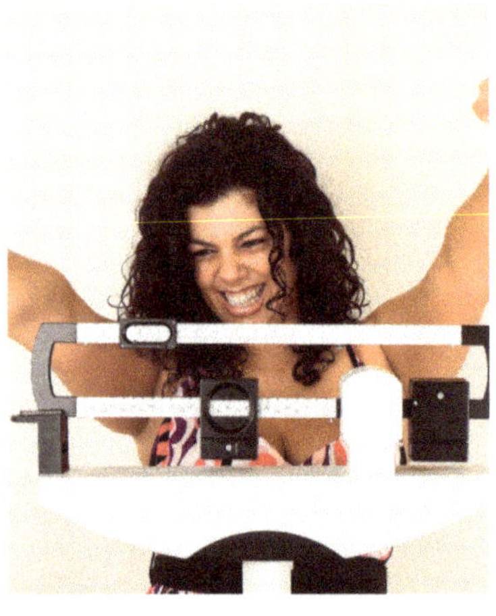

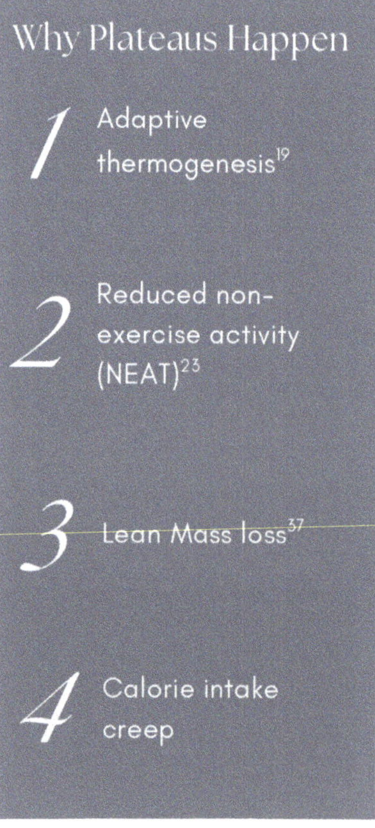

Why Plateaus Happen

Adaptive Thermogenesis

As body weight decreases, total daily energy expenditure decreases.

You burn fewer calories because:
- You weigh less
- You move a lighter body
- Resting metabolic rate declines

Additionally, adaptive thermogenesis may further reduce energy expenditure beyond what is predicted by weight loss alone.[19]

This is not damage, It is survival biology.

Reduced Non-Exercise Activity (NEAT)

Non-exercise activity thermogensis (NEAT) includes:
- Walking
- Fidgeting
- Postural movement
- Daily tasks

When calories do drop, spontaneous movement often decreases unconsciously.[23]

You may be moving less without realizing it.

Why Plateaus Happen

Lean Mass Lost

If muscle was lost earlier in the process, resting metabolic rate may be lower.[37]

Less muscle = lower baseline energy expenditure.

This reinforces why strength training is protective and necessary.

Calorie Intake Creep

Appetite suppression may be strong early on especially when starting a new health journey.

Over time, intake can increase slightly – even subtly.

Small increases matter when body size is smaller.

This is not failure.

It is human physiology adjusting.

What Not To Do

When the scale stalls, many women cut calories aggressively, skip protein, increase cardio excessively, or stop strength training due to fatigue.

These strategies increase lean mass loss and worsen metabolic adaptation.

More restriction is rarely the solution. Better structure is.

Hidden Calories - The Silent Weight Loss Saboteur

One of the most common reasons fat loss stalls, even on GLP-1, is unintentional calorie underestimation.

Research consistently shows that individuals underestimate caloric intake by 20-50%, particularly when eating restaurant meals.[13,29]

When your daily caloric intake target is around 1,500-1,700 calories, a single restaurant meal can quietly exceed half your day's energy needs.

Where Hidden Calories Lurk

1. **Salad Dressings** - a healthy salad can shift quickly:

- 2 tablespoons ranch 140-160 calories
- 2 tablespoons Caesar 150-180 calories

Many restaurants use 4-6 tablespoons unless specified. That can mean over 400 calories before protein and other toppings.

Dietitian Tip: Ask for dressing on the side and use 1-2 tablespoons intentionally.

Look for lower calorie versions when at home, or make your own!

2. **Cooking Oils** - restuarants prioritize flavor and texture, which means generous oil and butter use.
   Just one tablespoon oil is about 120 calories.

Pan seared meat and vegetables may contain 240-360 added calories without you even noticing.

Where Hidden Calories Lurk

3. **"Healthy" Bowls** - grain bowls often contain:

- 1-1.5 cups of rice or quinoa (200-330 calories)
- Added oil based sauces (150-250 calories)
- Nuts or seeds (100-200 calories)
- Avocado (120-240 calories)

Individually all of these are very healthy and great additions. But together with protein they can add up to a healthy bowl with over 1,000 calories easily.

Dietitian Tip: Limit higher calorie bowl options and stick to one grain, lots of vegetables, one protein, and one high fat item.

Or make your healthy bowl at home.

4. **Beverages** - anything but water can quickly add calories.

- Oat milk latte: 180-250 calories without sweetener
- Matcha: over 200 calories
- Alcoholic drinks: 100-300 calories

Alcoholic intake can also reduce dietary restraint later in the meal further incresing calorie creep.

Dietitian Tip: stick to water, unsweetened teas, coffees with splash of creamer, sparkling water, etc. Limit alcohol and avoid high sugar mixed drinks.

Where Hidden Calories Lurk

5. "Light" Menu Items

Menu labeling laws improved nutrition awareness but studies show that many restaurant meals still exceed stated calorie counts.[29]

Portions are often larger than standard serving sizes used in nutrition tracking apps.

Dietitian Tip: Eat at home (have I mentioned that yet?) If you regularly get a meal out, consider weighing these items at home and recalculating the calorie and nutrition content for better tracking.

Why This Matters More on GLP-1s?

When appetite is reduced, protein intake can already be borderline. If 400-600 hidden calories come from oil, dressing, beverages it can be easy to overeat calories and undereat protein and fiber.

How to Navigate Restaurants Without Obsessing?

1. Anchor Protein First – aim for 4 to 6 oz of grilled fish, chicken, steak, or tofu

2. Control Added Fats. Ask for:
   - Light oil
   - Sauce on the side
   - No butter finish

3. Choose **One** Energy-Dense Add-On
   - Alcohol
   - Creamy sauce
   - Fries
   - Dessert

Choose ONE. Not all four.

Plateau Troubleshooting

1. Protein Intake

Are you meeting your target?

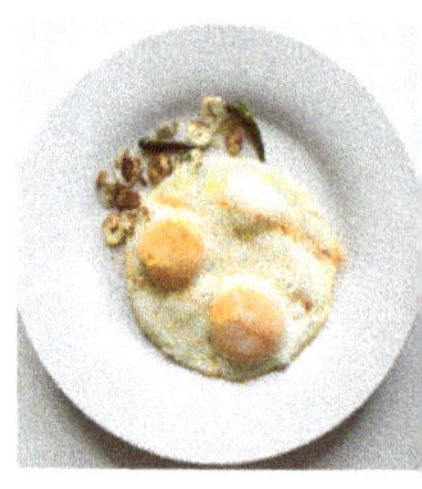

Inadequate protein intake increases lean mass loss and may reduce metabolic rate.[22]

If unsure, track intake for 3-5 days objectively to reassess how you are hitting your goals.

2. Strength Training

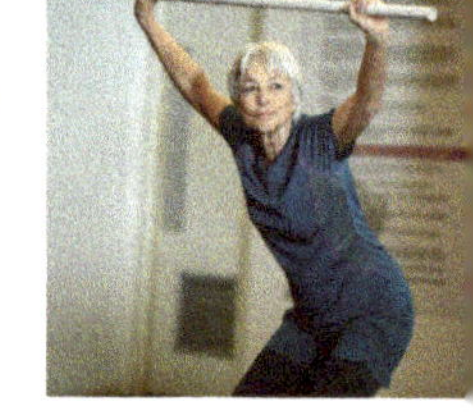

Are you getting 2-4 strength training sessions a week with progressive overload?

If workouts have become lighter or inconsistent, muscle stimulus may be insufficient.

Even 2 focused sessions per week matter.

3. Daily movement

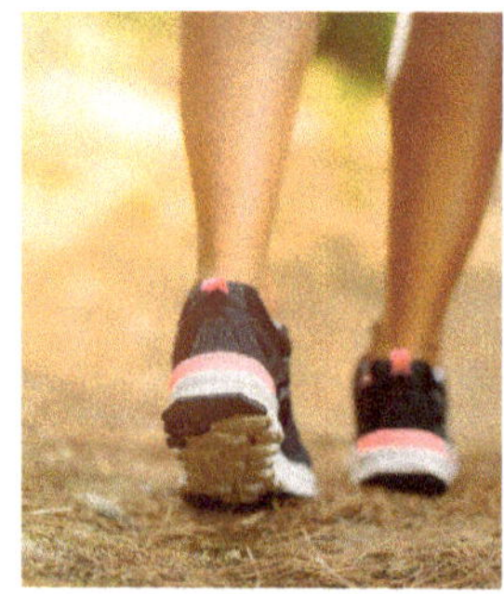

Check your average daily steps.

Has movement decreased lately?

A practical target is 7,000-10,000 steps per day.

4. Sleep

Sleep restriction alters hunger hormones and may impair fat loss.

Aim for 7-9 hours nightly.

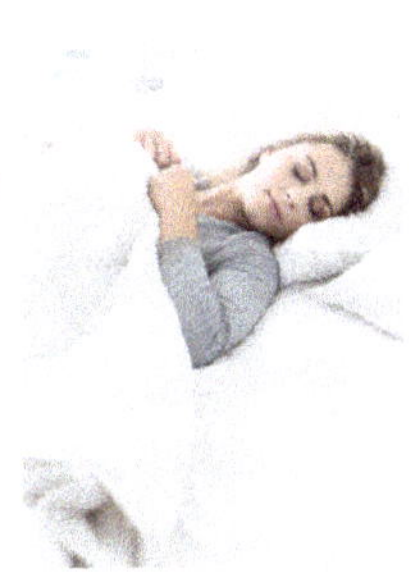

5. Rate of Loss So Far

If you have already lost significant weight, your energy needs are lower.

What worked at 180 pounds will not work at 150 pounds.

Calorie needs decrease as body mass decreases.

This is expected.

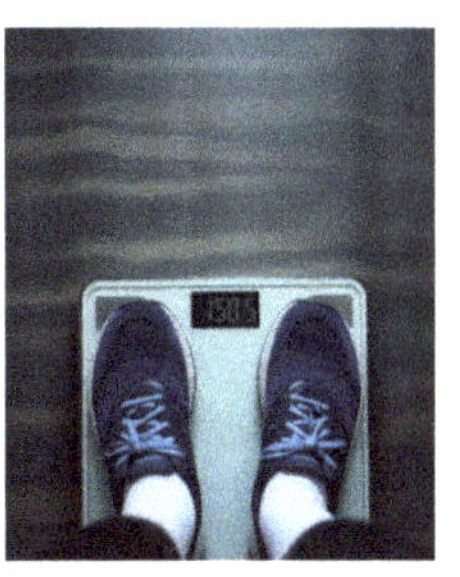

When Small Adjustments are Appropriate

If adherence is solid and plateau persists, options include:
- Slight protein increase
- Small calorie adjustments of 100-200 calories daily
- Increase daily steps modestly
- Review strength progression
- Evaluate medication dosing with provider

Avoid large swings.

Small adjustments can add up for success and prevent muscle loss.

Refeeds and Diet Breaks

In prolonged deficits, short diet breaks may help mitigate metabolic adaptation.[19]

This does not mean binge eating.

It means structured increase to estimated maintenace for 1-2 weeks while maintaining protein and strength training.

This approach may support training performance, reduce fatigue, and support metabolic rate.

If you have been eating 1,000-1,200 calories consistently, consider eating closer to 1,400-1,600 calories+ daily for a few weeks and beyond to shift metabolic rate.

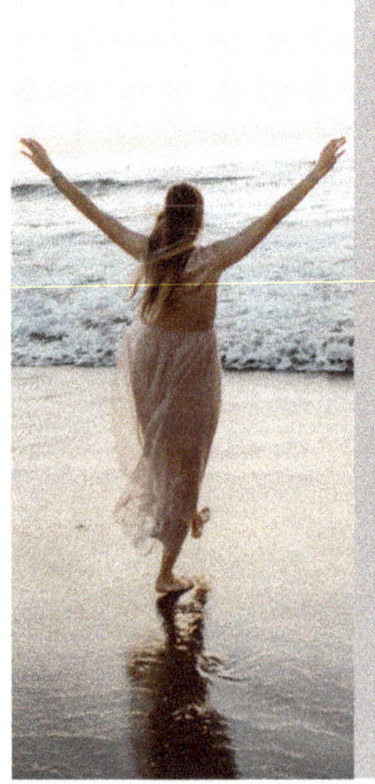

The Emotional Side of Plateaus

A stall often triggers:
- Fear of regain
- Urgency
- Overcorrection

But plateaus are part of every weight loss process, medicated or not.

Sustainable fat loss is not linear.

The body pauses before it changes again and removing fear and anxiety of plateaus will make for more sustainable change.

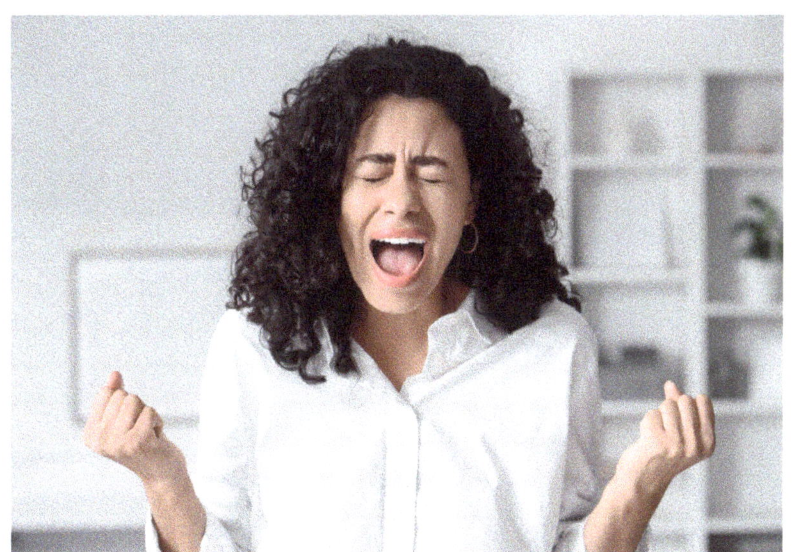

When to Reassess Goals

Sometimes a plataeu reflects that you are closer to your body's comfortable set point. Further loss may require greater precision, more time, and a reassessment of goals.

Health is not defined by the final 5 pounds.

Plateaus are physiological, not personal. The solution is structural refinement, not panic. GLP-1 medictions assist appetite control they do not eliminate metabolic adaptation.

Strategy always matter.

Plateau Checklist

1. Have I been tracking protein intake accurately?

2. Have I maintained strength training 2-4x per week?

3. Have I averaged at least 7,000 steps daily?

4. Have I slept at least 7 hours per night?

5. Have I avoided drastic calorie cuts?

08 Transition & Maintenance Blueprint

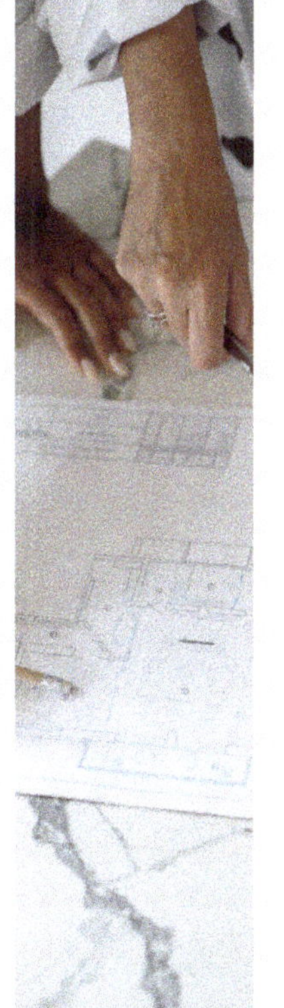

GLP-1 medications are powerful tools.

But they are not meant to replace skill, structure, or physiology.

Some individuals remain on these medications long term.
Others transition off for personal, financial, or medical reasons.

The question is not whether you stay on or off it.

The question is: **Have you built the foundation to maintain your results either way?**

What Happens When GLP-1 is Discontinued?

Research shows that after discontinuation of semaglutide, some weight regain is common if supportive lifestyle strategies are not maintained.[35]

When GLP-1 medication is withdrawn, appetite regulation returns to baseline physiology.

This is not failure.

It is biology reasserting itself.

If muscle mass was preserved during weight loss, resting energy expenditure may also be lower than before weight reduction.[19,37]

This combination - increased appetite + lower expenditure = creates vulnerability for regain.

Unless structure is in place.

The Three Pillars of Maintenace

Long-term success rests on three pillars:

1. Muscle preservation
2. Protein adequacy
3. Behavioral rhythm

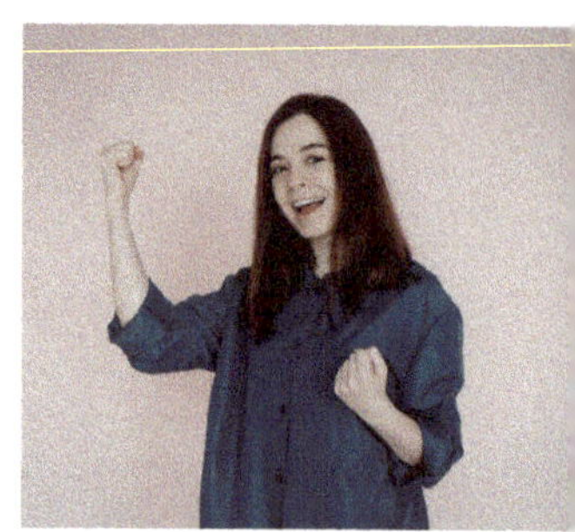

Pillar 1 - Muscle Is Your Metabolic Insurance

Lean muscle strongly influences resting metabolic rate.[37]

If strength training was consistent during weight loss, you have preserved metabolic capacity.

If it was not, rebuilding muscle becomes essential during transition.

Remember the minimum is 2 up to 4 sessions of progressive overload weekly.

Maintenance requires stimulus.

Muscle is metabolically active tissue, but only if you use it.

Pillar 2 - Protein as an Anchor Habit

During weight loss, higher protein intake preserves lean mass.[22]

During maintenance, protein remains protective.

A practical daily target is 0.7-1.0 grams per pound of body weight.

Protein will help:
- Improve satiety
- Stabilize blood sugar
- Supports recovery
- Reduces overeating risk

When appetite increases post-medication, protein becomes even more important.

Pillar 3 - Structured Eating Rhythm

GLP-1 therapy often reduces impulsive eating. Unfortunately too many clients I see have used this to eat too little and sporadically.

When transitioning off, hunger cues may return more strongly. If you did not put in place a solid eating schedule, it can be hard to adjust.

Instead of reaching emotionally, build structure now.

Example rhythm:
- 3 protein anchored meals (or 4 small meals)
- 1 planned high protein snack if needed (if only eating 3 meals)
- Consistent meal timing
- Daily hydration

Structure prevents reactive eating and can help minimize overating, especially when overeating is often on unhealthy food choices.

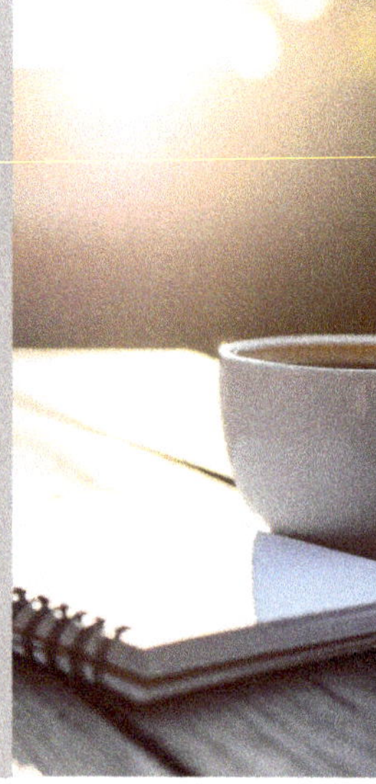

Gradual vs Abrupt Discontinuation

Any medication adjustment should be discussed with your prescribing provider.

In some cases, gradual tapering of GLP-1 may allow behavioral adaptation while appetite signals normalize.

During taper:
- Monitor hunger patterns
- Increase protein if appetite rises
- Maintain strength training
- Avoid panic restriction

Expect an Adjustment Phase

When transitioning off GLP-1, you may notice increased hunger, stronger food thoughts, larger portion tolerance.

This does not mean regain is ineveitable. It means appetite regulation has normalized.

Respond with protein first,
planned meals, mindful pacing,
and strength consistency.

Avoid skipping meals, over-restriction, and 'starting over' cycles.

How Much Regain is Normal?

Small weight fluctuations (3-5 pounds) during maintenance are common and reflect glycogen restoration, increased hydration, hormonal shifts.

This is not fat regain.

Fat regain is progressive and sustained upward trend over several weeks.

Monitor trends and don't spiral over normal weight fluctuations.

Reverse Dieting

Some individuals benefit from gradually increasing calorie intake toward estimated maintenance.

This can:
- Improve training performance
- Reduced fatigue
- Support metabolic adaptation recovery

A practical approach is to increase intake by 100-150 calories per week while keeping protein consistent and continuing workouts.

My Long-Term Maintenance Blueprint

Fill this out before transitioning

1. Goal weight range:

2. Protein floor (0.7-1.0 grams per pound goal weight):

3. Strength training days per week and schedule:

4. Average daily steps goal:

5. Meal structure plan:

6. Non-negotiable habits:

7. Action plan if weight increases more than 5 pounds:

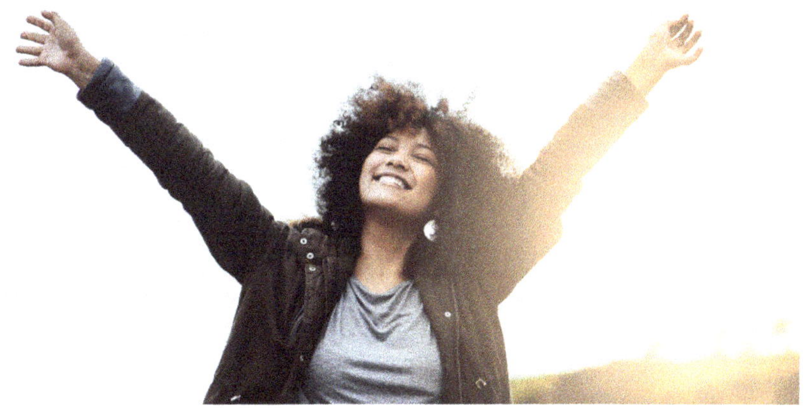

The Identity Shift

For some individuals with obesity as a chronic disease, long-term pharmacotherapy may be medically appropriate.

Obesity is a chronic, relapsing condition.

This is no moral superiority in discontinuing medication.

The goal is health stability.

Discuss options with your providor.

The final and most important shift:
You are not 'someone on medication trying to lose weight.'

You are someon who:
- Prioritizes their health
- Prioritizes protein
- Strength trains consistently
- Maintains structure
- Monitors trends calmly

Medication may have opened the door, your habits keep it open.

A Final Letter to You

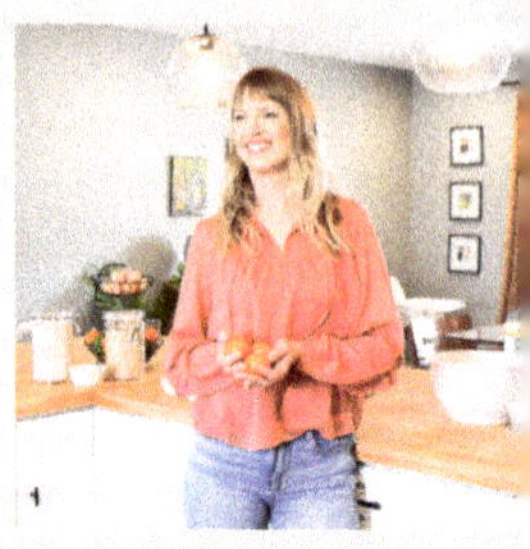

If you have read this far, I want you to pause for a moment.

Not to think about your weight.
Not to calculate calories.
Not to evaluate your progress.

Just pause.
Because choosing to understand your body instead of fighting it is not a small decision.

It is a shift.

For years, you may have been told that weight loss is about willpower. That hunger is weakness. That struggle means you are failing.

But biology is not a moral issue. Hunger is not a character flaw. Plateaus are not punishment. Weight regain is not proof that you are broken.

Your body is adaptive, protective, and intelligent.

GLP-1 medications may have helped quiet the noise. They may have created space. They may have allowed you to expereince what a regulated appetite feels like.

But medication is not your discipline. It is not your identity. It is not your worth.
The real work was never just about the scale.

It was about:

- Learning to prioritize protein even when appetite was low
- Strength training when the excitement faded
- Building structure instead of chasing motivation
- Choosing consistency over intensity

Those are skills.
Skills are portable.

Whether you remain on medication long term or transition off, the foundation you build is what protects your progress.

Muscle protects metabolism.
Protein protects muscle.
Structure protects behavior.
Self-awareness protects everything.

There will be weeks and days when things feel easy. There may be weeks and days when hunger returns louder than expected. There may be moments when the scale moves in ways you do not like.

Respond with data, not drama.
Adjust. Do not abandon.
Refine. Do not restart.

The process was never about shrinking yourself. It was about stabilizing your health. If this book has given you clarity, structure, or even a small reducation in shame, then it has done its job.

Anna, RD

BONUS - 7 Day Meal Plan

This meal plan provides approximately 1,600 calories per day
120-140 grams protein daily
28-40 grams of fiber daily

Portions can be adjusted to meet individual needs.

Day	Breakfast	Lunch	Dinner	Snack
Monday	Greek Power Yogurt Bowl 1 cup nonfat greek yogurt ½ cup blueberries 1 tbsp chia seeds ¼ cup high-fiber granola 1 scoop collagen or whey mixed in 400 cal, 40 g pro	Grilled Chicken & Quinoa Bowl 4 oz grilled chicken breast ½ cup cooked quinoa 1 cup roasted broccoli 1 tbsp olive oil Lemon + herbs 450 cal, 38 g pro	Salmon, Sweet Potato, & Green Beans 4 oz baked salmon with lemon + herbs 150 g roasted sweet potato 1 cup green beans 500 cal, 35 g pro	Apple + 2 tbsp natural peanut butter 250 cal, 8 g pro
Tuesday	Protein Oatmeal ½ cup oats 1 scoop vanilla whey protein powder 1 tbsp ground flaxseed ½ banana cinnamon 400 cal, 35 g protein	Turkey & Avocado Wrap high fiber tortilla 4 oz sliced turkey breast ¼ avocado Shredded lettuce/spinach Mustard or low cal dressing Baby carrots 450 cal, 35 g pro	Ground Beef Stir Fry 4 oz 93% ground beef 1 cup mixed vegetables ¾ cup cauliflower rice ½ cup jasmine rice 2 tbsp soy sauce Hot sauce to flavor 500 cal, 35 g pro	1 cup low fat cottage cheese + ½ cup pineapple or fruit of choice 220 cal, 28 g pro
Wed	Egg White & Veggie Scramble 1 whole egg 1 cup egg whites spinach, mushrooms, peppers or other veggies of choice 1 slice whole grain toast 400 cal, 38 g pro	Tuna & White Bean Salad 1 can tuna in water ½ cup white beans 1 cup+ arugula or spinach ½ cup cherry tomatoes 1 tbsp olive oil fresh lemon juice or apple cider vinegar 450 cal, 40 g pro	Chicken Fajita Bowl 4 oz grilled chicken with fajita seasoning ½ cup black beans ½ cup rice 1 cup cooked peppers + onions salsa/hot sauce 450 cal, 35 g pro	Protein smoothie with 1 scoop whey, 1 cup unsweetened almond milk, ½ cup frozen berries, 1 tbsp peanut butter 300 cal, 30 g pro

BONUS - 7 Day Meal Plan

Day	Breakfast	Lunch	Dinner	Snack
Thurs	Chia Protein Pudding 2 tbsp chia seeds ¾ cup nonfat greek yogurt ½ scoop protein powder ½ cup raspberries 400 cal, 35 g pro	Shrimp Power Salad 5 oz cooked shrimp 1+ cup mixed greens ½ sliced cucumber ½ cup chickpeas 1 tbsp olive oil + 2 tsp vinegar 450 cal, 40 g pro	Turkey Meatballs & Zucchini Noodles 4 oz turkey meatballs ½ cup marinara 1 cup zoodles ½ cup whole wheat pasta 500 cal, 35 g pro	High protein snack bar with more than 15 g protein around 200 cal, 15+ g pro
Fri	Protein Pancakes 1 serving protein pancake mix with ½ cup egg whites ¼ cup berries to top 2 tbsp low sugar syrup 400 cal, 35 g pro	Chicken Caesar Salad 5 oz grilled chicken breast 1+ cup romaine lettuce 2 tbsp light caesar dressing 2 tbsp parmesan ¼ cup chickpeas 450 cal, 45 g pro	Baked Cod + Lentils 5 oz baked cod with lemon + herbs ½ cup lentils cooked 1 cup roasted asparagus 550 cal, 40 g pro	1 cup edamame 190 cal, 17 g pro
Sat	Cottage Cheese Bowl 1 cup low fat cottage cheese ½ cup strawberries 1 tbsp almond butter 1 tbsp hemp seeds 400 cal, 35 g pro	Ground Turkey Taco Bowl 4 oz ground turkey with fajita seasoning ½ cup black beans 1 cup shredded lettuce ½ cup pico de gallo ½ cup rice 500 cal, 38 g pro	Grilled Chicken + Roasted Brussel Sprouts + Baked Potato 5 oz grilled chicken 1 1/2 cup roasted Brussels sprouts 1 tsp olive oil 1 small baked potato 450 cal, 40 g pro	1 pear + 1 oz almonds 250 cal, 6 g pro
Sun	Overnight Protein Oats ½ cup oats ¾ cup nonfat Greek yogurt ½ scoop protein powder ½ cup blueberries 1 tbsp chia seeds 400 cal, 35 g pro	Salmon Salad Plate 4 oz baked salmon ½ cup farro 1+ cup arugula or spinach ½ cup roasted carrots 1 tbsp olive oil 500 cal, 35 g pro	Steak Bowl 4 oz lean steak 1 1/2 cup roasted cauliflower 1 tsp olive oil ½ cup quinoa 450 cal, 35 g pro	Protein shake + 1 small apple 250 cal, 30 g pro

References

1. American College of Sports Medicine. (2016). Exercise and fluid replacement. *Medicine & Science in Sports & Exercise*, 48(3), 543-568.
2. Babault N, et al. (2015). Pea protein supplementation promotes muscle thickness gains during resistance training: A double-blind, randomized, placebo-controlled clinical trial. *Journal of the International Society of Sports Nutrition*, 12(1), 3.
3. Bleich SN, et al. (2015). Calorie changes in chain restaurant menu items after implementation of calorie labeling. *American Journal of Preventative Medicine*, 53(6), 809-813.
4. Blundell J, et al. (2017). Effects of once-weekly semaglutide on appetite, energy intake, control of eating, and food preference. *Diabetes, Obesity, and Metabolism*, 19(9), 1242-1251.
5. Boirie Y, et al. (1997). Slow and fast dietary proteins differently modulate postprandial protein accretion. *Proceedings of the National Academy of Sciences*, 94(26), 14930-14935.
6. Fothergill E et al. (2016). Persistent metabolic adaptation 6 years after "The Biggest Loser" competition. *Obesity*.
7. Ha E, & Zemel MB. (2003). Functional properties of whey, whey components, and essential amino acids: Mechanisms underlying health benefits for active people. *Journal of Nutritional Biochemistry*, 14(5), 251-258.
8. Hall KD, et al. (2016). Energy expenditure and body composition changes after an isocaloric ketogenic diet in overweight and obese men. *American Journal of Clinical Nutrition*, 104(2), 324-333).
9. Harris L, et al. (2018). Intermittent fasting interventions for treatment of overweight and obesity. *JBI Database System Rev.*
10. Holst JJ. (2007). The physiology of glucagon-like peptide 1. *Physiological Reviews*, 87(4), 1409-1439.
11. Jastreboff AM, et al. (2022). Tirzepatide once weekly for the treatment of obesity. *New England Journal of Medicine*, 387, 205-216.
12. Leidy HJ, et al. (2015). The role of protein in weight loss and maintenance. *American Journal of Clinical Nutrition*, 101(6), 1320S-1329S.
13. Lichtman SW, et al. (1992) Discrepancy between self-reported and actual caloric intake and exercise in obese subjects. *New England Journal of Medicine*, 327(27), 1893-1898.
14. Lowe DA et al. (2020). Effects of time-restricted eating on weight loss and metabolic disease risk factors. *JAMA International Medicine*.
15. Loucks AB. (2003). Energy availability, not body fatness, regulates reproductive function in women. *Exercise Sports Review.*
16. Mamerow MM, et al. (2014) Dietary protein distribution positively influences muscle protein synthesis. *Journal of Nutrition*, 144(6), 876-880.
17. Messina M. (2018). Soy and Health Update: Evaluation of the Clinical and Epidemiologic Literature. *Nutrients*, 10(7), 857.
18. Morton RW, et al. (2018). A systematic review, meta-analysis and meta-regression of the effect of protein supplementation on resistance training-induced gains in muscle mass and strength in healthy adults. *British Journal of Sports Medicine*, 52(6), 376-384.
19. Muller MJ & Bosy-Westphal A. (2013). Adaptive thermogenesis with weight loss. *Obesity*, 23(4), 712-719.
20. Norton LE, & Layman DK. (2006). Leucine regulates translation initiation of protein synthesis in skeletal muscle after exercise. *The Journal of Nutrition*, 136(2), 533S-537S.
21. Oikawa SY, et al. (2020). Whey protein but not collagen peptides stimulate acute and longer-term muscle protein synthesis. *The American Journal of Clinical Nutrition*, 111(3), 708-718.
22. Pasiakos SM, et al. (2013). Effects of high-protein diets on fat-free mass and muscle protein synthesis following weight loss: a randomized controlled trial. *FASEB Journal*, 27(9), 3837-3847.
23. Rosenbaum M, & Leibel RL. (2010). Adaptive thermogenesis in humans. *International Journal of Obesity*, 34(S1), S47-S55.
24. Schoenfeld BJ, et al. (2013). The effect of protein timing on muscle strength and hypertrophy: A meta-analysis. *Journal of the International Society of Sports Nutrition*, 10(1), 53.
25. Shaw G, et al. (2017). Vitamin C-enriched gelatin supplementation before intermittent activity augments collagen synthesis. *The American Journal of Clinical Nutrition*, 105(1), 136-143.
26. Shirreffs SM, & Sawka MN. (2011). Fluid and electrolyte needs for training, competition, and recovery. *Journal of Sports Science*, 29(supl), S39-S46.
27. Sutton EF et al. (2018). Early time-restricted feeding improves insulin sensitivity. Cellular Metabolism.
28. Tang JE, et al., (2009). Ingestion of whey hydrolysate, casein, or soy protein isolate: Effects on mixed muscle protein synthesis at rest and following resistance exercise. *Journal of Applied Physiology*, 107(3), 987-992.
29. Urban LE, et al. (2011). Accuracy of stated energy contents of restaurant foods. *JAMA*, 306(3), 287-293.
30. U.S. Food and Drug Administration. (2018). Menu labeling requirements.
31. Varady KA (2011). Intermittent versus daily caloric restriction: which diet regimen is more effective for weight loss? *Obesity Review*, 12(7), 593-601.
32. Weinheimer EM, et al. (2010). A systematic review of the separate and combined effects of energy restriction and exercise on fat-free mass in middle-aged and older adults: implications for sarcopenic obesity. *Journal of the American Diabetic Association*, 110(7), 1062-1074.
33. Westcott WL. (2012). Resistance training is medicine: Effects on health. *Current Sports Medicine Reports*, 11(4), 209-216.
34. Wilding JPH, et al. (2021) Once-weekly semaglutide in adults with overweight or obesity. *New England Journal of Medicine*, 384, 989-1002.
35. Wilding JPH, et al. (2022) Weight regain and cardiometabolic effect after withdrawal of semaglutide. *Diabetes, Obesity, and Metabolism*, 24(8), 1553-1564.
36. Wilkinson MJ, et al. (2020). Ten-hour time-restricted eating reduces weight and improves cardiometabolic health. *Cellular Metabolism*, 31(1), 92-104.
37. Wolfe RR. (2006). The underappreciated role of muscle in health and disease. *American Journal of Clinical Nutrition*, 84(3), 475-482.